Reviews for *Bui*

MW00937197

"*Burnout in Healthcare: A Guide to Addressing the Epidemic* provides an evidence-supported overview of clinician burnout, its causes and manifestations, as well as the consequences for everyone who touches the healthcare system. Its focus on solutions at both the organizational and individual levels will help clinicians and leaders better understand how to grapple with this serious issue—and especially important—with where to start. Everyone who works in clinical care or leads those who do needs to read this book."

— Diane W. Shannon, MD, MPH, writer, coach, and co-author of *Preventing Physician Burnout: Curing the Chaos and Returning Joy to the Practice of Medicine*

"Dr. Kurapati has written a concise and valuable guide to recognize and address burnout among medical professionals. A must-read for all physicians, nurses, and medical staff who strive to preserve their passion and sanity in the face of a relentless medical-industrial complex."

— David J. Naiman, MD, author of *Jake, Lucid Dreamer* and *Didn't Get Frazzled*

"As a nurse, I can fully identify with the concept of burnout. I believe this book by Dr. Kurapati is a great resource for anyone in the healthcare field. He shares valuable insights about this growing problem and suggests practical ways that healthcare providers and administrators can combat it head-on."

— Mandy Lawrence, registered nurse and author

"Dr. Kurapati has the rare skill of being a physician and a skilled written communicator. He demonstrates his humanism with this guide to preventing and/or escaping burnout, an epidemic among physicians today. Aside from understanding the causes and symptoms of burnout, Dr. Kurapati provides actionable items so that the reader can take away real skills from his book. This should be mandatory reading for anyone in healthcare, ranging from those in administration to physicians and other medical professionals."

— Dr. Nancy Yen Shipley, Orthopedic surgeon, speaker, and team physician for the U.S. Ski & Snowboard team

"If you feel like you aren't on your 'A' game, it might be because you're burned out but don't realize it. *Burnout in Healthcare* will give you the answers you seek and help you get back to your 'A' game again."

— Dr. Cory S. Fawcett, author of *Prescription for Financial Success*

"*Burnout in Healthcare: A Guide to Addressing the Epidemic* can serve as an excellent primer for individuals to learn how to recognize early signs of burnout. Dr. Kurapati's research explains that a multi-pronged effort requiring "conscious choices" at the individual, organizational, and policy making levels can achieve significant improvements in professional satisfaction as well as in the quality of healthcare delivered. For medical schools, hospital systems, and policy makers, the book is a valuable tool for understanding how to initiate the cultural paradigm shift needed to change the course of the burnout epidemic facing the healthcare industry."

— Dr. Carina Hopen, Family Physician, Certified Health
Coach, and former U.S. Naval Flight Surgeon

"*Burnout in Healthcare* provides a framework to consider and a comprehensive discussion on ways to mitigate this threat to providing the healthcare we all desire and need."

— Simon G. Talbot, MD, Attending Surgeon, Brigham
and Women's Hospital and Associate Professor,
Harvard Medical School

BURNOUT IN HEALTHCARE

BURNOUT IN HEALTHCARE

A GUIDE TO ADDRESSING THE EPIDEMIC

Rajeev Kurapati MD, MBA

To my fellow physicians, nurses, and medical staff who travel this professional journey with me. Your role is the most demanding as you field the front lines in patient care and treatment in this complicated medical-industrial complex.

You're devoted to helping your patients. But who's helping you?

Table of Contents

Introduction

Patients enter a hospital or clinic for one reason—they're looking for relief. This might come in the form of a diagnosis, a cure, or support and comfort for an incurable illness. To achieve this, two ingredients are essential: care and connection.

Imagine a hospital or a doctor's office where these critical factors are lacking. Healthcare providers might be physically present, but they're emotionally withdrawn and exhausted. Rather than engaging fully with patients and staff, they go through their days by rote habit, lacking passion and attention to detail. In this scenario, everyone suffers. Right now, this is exactly what's happening to medical staff in many healthcare organizations.

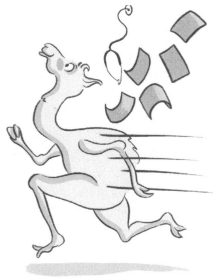

If you've found your way to this book, you're already familiar with this phenomenon. Burnout is a serious issue occurring at both an individual and organization level, and it calls for our immediate attention.

⸻

It's an exciting time to be in the *business* of healthcare, but for the medical professional—a nurse, doctor, or other care practitioner— it's becoming more and more stressful to keep up with expectations.

I've been practicing hospital medicine since 2008, and over the last decade I've seen many of my talented, high-achieving colleagues become shells of their former selves or exit the profession altogether. The balancing act of staying true to their patients' best interests and being subservient to rising pressures from regulators, policy makers, and insurance industries is driving practitioners beyond the tipping point—resulting in the breakdown of their resiliency.

Since the turn of the century, the healthcare profession has undergone dramatic changes, growing more advanced, faster paced, and increasingly complicated. This forward progress has pushed the limits of science to spectacular heights and saved many lives. We've bettered the treatment of diseases by standardizing protocols, implementing checklists to prevent medical errors, and improving proper antiseptic techniques. Technology has expanded the scale of medical research and made communication between patients and care providers easier.

Yet alongside these revolutionary benefits, we've also begun to see some undesirable consequences of the digitization of medicine.

Large-scale implementation of electronic health records, for instance, has made access to health information easier but added more work for already overloaded medical professionals. It's put the physician, nurse, and social worker into a mode of constant data entry. This combines with other existing pressures—like the urgency to keep costs down and the relentless drive for both patient accessibility and quality of care.

The result of these mounting expectations—coupled with a lack of proper self-care and meager organizational attention to care providers' well-being—is burnout.

Medical staff at all levels report widespread dissatisfaction and work-life imbalance. In turn, this perpetuates a cycle of detrimental outcomes. Staff burnout is associated with lower patient satisfaction and thus poor patient experience, as well as higher costs to health systems. This is then reflected in a shortage of healthcare workers (as practitioners leave the profession early), furthering the strain on those who stay.

For most healthcare workers, a career in medicine is driven by the desire to help others. Yet more and more physicians and nurses report feeling like the joy of medicine is gone. Unfortunately, many healthcare providers are already burned out before they can put the pieces together.

⸺⸙⸺

With this book, I set out to explore the nature of burnout, its many forms and symptoms, and ultimately its solutions. I spent months talking with physicians, nurses, and other care practitioners around the country (their names have been changed to maintain ano-nymity), and I drew input from their experiences and feedback. In addition, I dug into research by experts at Mayo Clinic and other organizations about the unique ways healthcare workers experience burnout, as well as how the profession is set up to exacerbate burn-out's causes and symptoms. I spoke with doctors who *don't* seem to be impacted by burnout to learn what they're doing differently. Then I synthesized all of that information here—creating a quick, informative guide addressing burnout for healthcare practitioners.

Burnout doesn't have a quick fix or a pill to swallow to ease the symptoms. Instead, it requires conscious choices to change both your physical environment and your inner world to find the free-dom you're looking for.

In the ensuing chapters, I explain how to recognize burnout and discuss its causes. Then I explore methods for addressing it—both at the organizational and individual levels. This book leads readers through techniques for developing resilience that can help create a stronger sense of satisfaction and fulfillment in the workplace and beyond.

You may not be in a position to make huge changes in your life or within your healthcare organization. Even so, there's still plenty for you to gain from this book, including practical, evidence-based strategies to help prevent future burnout, tackle it if you see the symptoms, and restore joy to your practice of caregiving—or even life itself.

—∞∞—

"Burnout is the sum total of hundreds and thousands of tiny betrayals of purpose, each one so minute that it hardly attracts notice."

— RICHARD GUNDERMAN

CHAPTER 1

Burnout: A Knotty Process

Burnout is going to impact different care providers in different ways. Let's start by taking a look at Sonia, a highly regarded kidney specialist who prides herself on her passion for her work. In her 24 years as a physician, her patients and their families have always been quick to point out her compassionate care and attention to detail. She not only puts in extra time tending to patients as they come in, but also in following up with them after discharge. Her colleagues love her, too, and she's well respected by nurses, other physicians, and administrative staff at her Arizona hospital.

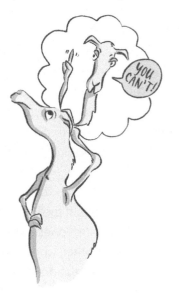

On the outside, the 53-year-old is a shining example of the perfect medical specialist. But what her patients and colleagues—and even Sonia herself—don't realize is that she's falling apart.

For many years, Sonia looked forward to work. As she woke up each morning and got ready for the day, her interactions with patients were a powerful fuel that drove her dedication and ambition. But lately, Sonia has found herself gripped by a terrible feeling of dread. It starts on Sunday nights as she anticipates going to work. The feeling blooms into anxiety and overwhelm by Monday morning. She's able to grit her teeth and knuckle her way through the week, but as the hours of each day progress, she begins to exhibit physical manifestations of her inner stress. Within moments of interacting with her patients, she's suddenly battling an upset stomach, her throat dries up, and she's surprised by the urge to slip out the doors of the hospital into the parking lot.

Connecting with patients—which used to come naturally—has become exasperating. Sonia's interactions at work, and then later at home, leave her feeling drained. Even the act of making minor, insignificant decisions is distressing, and she criticizes herself for losing her edge.

Every afternoon, Sonia is struck by a profound feeling of restlessness. For a woman who's been driven by passion and purpose since she was a child, this new state creates a lot of guilt. She's never been in a situation where she's felt this inadequate. The guilt compounds, adding to her stress.

And when it's time to leave the hospital each evening, there's no relief. Throughout the year, Sonia has ended her work days as a physician and transitioned into an equally intense role: a caregiver to her elderly mother, whose condition continues to decline. Sonia can see there's no real down time to recharge and nurture herself, but what can she do? Her patients need her. Her mother needs her, too.

Late at night, despite trying to briefly unwind at home after the day's long list of tasks has been tended to, Sonia struggles with insomnia that leaves her dragging during daylight hours. As months pass like this, Sonia begins gaining weight and even losing some of her hair. Tired and demoralized, she first writes off her symptoms as menopause or aging, but then she begins to wonder if something else is wrong. She even makes an appointment with a therapist, who prescribes an anti-depressant. Sonia dutifully takes the pills each morning for a few months, but they don't offer the relief she's looking for.

Sonia begins reflecting on her situation in earnest. She knows something has to change, but she isn't sure what. She doesn't know it just yet, but she's in the throes of burnout.

—⊶⊷—

Burnout is a knotty process. It happens slowly, slowly, slowly—and then suddenly, it's upon you. It isn't exactly that burnout accelerates, but that we often ignore or misunderstand the signs and symptoms until they coalesce dramatically into hopelessness. What's especially tricky is that many of burnout's markers are easily masked because they mimic so many other psychological maladies. This is a key reason why the healthcare workplace is in a burnout epidemic.

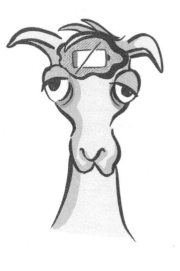

In the United states, more than 42% of physicians report they're currently experiencing or have recently experienced burnout, according to Medscape's 2018 Physician Burnout and Depression Report, which interviewed 15,543 physicians across 29 specialties. And this isn't limited to the United States. Around the globe, countries such as Germany, Hungary, the United Kingdom, Portugal, and likely many more are seeing increases in burnout across a wide range of healthcare specialties as well.

In 2008, the European General Practice Research Network (EGPRN) Burnout Study Group, which interviewed nearly 1,400 family doctors in 12 countries, found numbers similar to the United States: 43% of participating physicians showed an elevated degree of emotional exhaustion, 35% exhibited high levels of depersonalization, and 32% demonstrated a sense of low personal and professional achievement.

Burnout isn't only plaguing end-stage-career physicians, either. The highest concentration of those reporting burnout in the U.S. were ages 45 to 54—healthcare providers who were still right in the middle of their careers. It turns out burnout also brings along some other unsavory friends. Of respondents in the Medscape report, 70% were also experiencing depression. In worst-case scenarios, untreated burnout has even been shown to drive physicians to suicide.

Nurse burnout is on the rise too—one study found as many as 43% of nurses and other caregivers were experiencing the emotional exhaustion indicative of burnout. Many other kinds of care providers, including social workers, medical assistants, and even those who act as caregivers to ailing family members or a child with a disability can easily fall victim to burnout.

Beyond the impact burnout carries on a healthcare professional's well-being, the financial losses related to burnout are staggering for medical institutions as a whole. A 2017 Stanford report estimated that physician burnout costs the United States anywhere from $2.9 to $5 billion every year due to the expense of replacing physicians who are leaving their jobs earlier in their careers. Adding to this figure is the reality that burned-out doctors often contribute substandard patient care. At best, this leaves patients dissatisfied or outraged, and the organization's bottom line suffers. At worst, the consequences for patients can be life altering.

Of course, burnout isn't limited to healthcare—it impacts individuals in industries from teaching to finance. While a majority of the practical steps here could be applied no matter what an individual does for a living, the scope of this book addresses burnout in the healthcare field, specifically.

—⚬❀⚬—

"The unexamined life is not worth living."

— SOCRATES

CHAPTER 2

Recognizing Burnout

C arol, a pediatric nurse who's been working for a large Midwest hospital for more than two decades, is accustomed to receiving kudos for being highly organized, compassionate, and competent. "Call Carol" is a go-to phrase the other nurses use when things on the floor are overwhelming. At 45 years old and the mother of 12-year-old twins, she's beloved by her young patients, and their happy faces are one of the great rewards of her work.

But over time she's noticed she has difficulty prioritizing tasks and keeping track of simple information. She gets distracted easily and forgets where she's supposed to be going next. She finds herself avoiding colleagues she normally loves to chat with and rushing through appointments instead. She pursues a medical work up, but when it comes back clean, Carol is at a loss. It takes her several months to realize she isn't losing her mind—she's burned out.

For others, the signs of burnout can be less obvious. Jack, a 58-year-old Boston-based psychiatrist who's been practicing for close to 30 years, treats numerous patients with various mental illnesses while working for a big medical system—he believes he's already well versed in the signs of burnout. Yet he doesn't think too much of his own growing urge to have a drink or three after arriving home for the day, or his slowly building irritability with minor details at work. He shrugs off his wife's concern that he seems more tired and cranky than usual.

It isn't until he notices how averse he's become to going to work morning after morning that Jack allows himself to consider something might be wrong. "I've been quick to interrupt my patients," he admits to me. "I have an all-around impatience—I've even snapped at my staff a few times." Coupled with what feels like an utter loss of his sense of humor, Jack can sense that something isn't right, but he isn't sure where to start.

When he blows up at an administrative assistant over a minor error in an uncharacteristic moment of rage, he realizes, "After helping others with burnout for years, I finally see I'm experiencing it myself."

Hiding Behind the Smoke Screen

One reason burnout can be so insidious is that even many medical professionals don't recognize the signs or ask for help until they're at the point where they need to quit their career altogether. In the Medscape National Physician Burnout & Depression Report for 2018, only about 9% of the physicians interviewed reported seeking professional help when facing symptoms of burnout. Even then, psychiatric assessment may not always be the right kind of help. Here's why: psychiatric evaluation may not reveal the problem. A psychiatrist is likely to speak with a patient for a few minutes and may prescribe counseling, an antidepressant, or other psychotropic medication based on a description of prominent burnout symptoms, which only masks the problem.

Adding to the complication, burnout manifests in plenty of different ways. While it may present as depression or anxiety, it can also exacerbate any number of other underlying psychiatric illnesses, such as bipolar disorder or borderline personality disorder. Despite this, burnout alone doesn't fit in any diagnostic criteria for established mental illnesses. In fact, there's not yet specific diagnostic criteria for burnout in DSM-5 (the fifth edition of the Diagnostic and Statistical Manual for Mental Disorders), which represents the most comprehensive and widely used information currently available for clinical diagnosis of mental disorders.

What Burnout Really Feels Like

Recognizing early warning signs of burnout is difficult, but the end result is the same in all cases: You become what we'll call **DEF**. When in burnout, you experience **D**epersonalization, **E**motional exhaustion, and decreased **F**unction at work. Another way to look at this is that you become cynical, exhausted, and perform poorly.

For healthcare professionals, burnout may translate to a day-to-day experience of feeling like you're rushing from one patient or procedure to the next without any sense of fulfillment. For caregivers, it may feel more like you're trapped in a cycle of all work, no satisfaction.

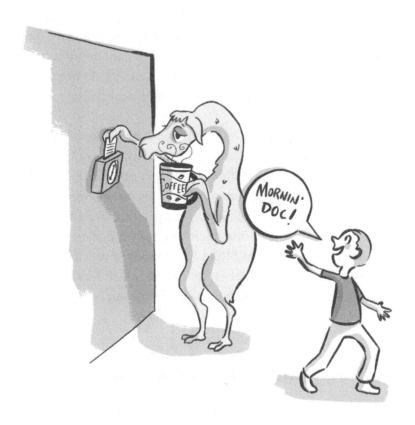

In order to determine if you're suffering from burnout, here are two simple steps to help you make that call.

Step 1: Answer this question:

Do you often feel like "I can't do this anymore," even after an initial period of adaptation to your job?

If you answered yes, go on to the next step.

Step 2: Look out for the following symptoms:

1. You have less patience with others than you used to.

2. You feel physically exhausted right at the beginning of your workday.

3. You habitually feel like you're making errors of judgement despite adequate training.

If you answered yes to these three questions, you're likely burned out.

The above feelings may culminate in a host of symptoms, including sleepless nights, mindless preoccupations, becoming socially withdrawn, nervousness, irritability, avoidance of exercise and social interaction, and craving junk food.

If you did answer yes to those questions, you aren't alone. Understanding you're experiencing burnout means you can take actionable steps toward solutions.

Am I Stressed Out or Burned Out?

Burnout is an individual, subjective experience that happens in the space between your ears. To determine if you're experiencing burnout, it's important to distinguish between regular job-associated stress and actual burnout.

When reality doesn't match our expectations, we experience stress. Workplace stress is not uncommon for physicians and other healthcare workers. It can come from many directions and may be the result of too many expectations, mounting pressures, or external factors, like too little staffing.

While stress is often destructive, we can't ignore its ability to push us to optimal alertness and performance. The existence of stress hormones is an incredible biological adaptation that provides us with the ability to deal with high-intensity situations—imbuing us with the power of resiliency and helping us adapt to whatever our jobs (or lives) may throw our way.

While small amounts of stress can propel us forward, as a constant condition, chronic stress becomes harmful. To manage it, one of the most helpful things we can do is identify specific problem areas and take concrete steps to address the source.[1] While some types of stress may be difficult to manage, in most cases, stress is easy to recognize.

Burnout is a different animal. It's the great imitator, so we may not recognize it for what it is. For instance, you may be a high-performing leader or a well-loved team player, doing all the things that count as being "successful" and yet, after many years of following your passion, you may suddenly feel that nothing you do is meaningful anymore. You may feel unmotivated, unchallenged, or bored at a job you were once very enthusiastic about. You

---

1   Notice I mention "managing" stress, not "eliminating" it. You can never fully eliminate stress (nor would you want to), as it's a biological mechanism that enables us to adapt to changing situations in life. By managing stress to an optimal level, however, we function most effectively.

don't want to quit the job you spent years training for, but at the same time you dread (or feel restless) going to work day after day. Waiting to see if this feeling will pass only seems to make it worse.

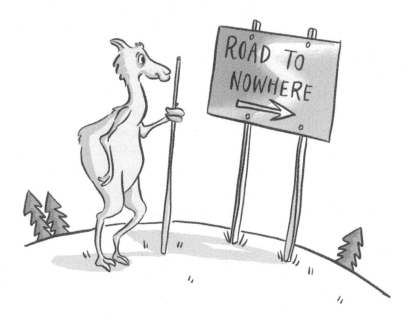

It's important to remember these feelings aren't occurring because you're less competent or capable or that you're lacking in some way. You're still the right person for the job, but your energy and enthusiasm are tapped out because they haven't been nurtured and balanced.

It's not uncommon to experience stress if you're early in your career, where it may take time to adjust to new responsibilities, a new workplace culture, and the demands of working full time. In this case, initial jitters typically melt away with experience and adaptation.

If you find that a set of new job responsibilities doesn't match your core competencies—what you like to do and what you're good at—you may experience dissatisfaction and stress, but that's not necessarily burnout. For example, I'm at my best in an acute and intense environment. You'll see me thriving when I'm running between hospital floors handling cardiac events and other critical care crises. Acute care is my core competency; I become bored and restless in a more routine patient care setting. Another person, however, might feel better working in a clinic where patients come to them by way of a predetermined schedule—such as an endocrinologist or a rheumatologist. This person would become stressed doing my job, and I'd stress out doing theirs. If you find that your job is causing you stress, you may want to explore other roles within your field that are a better match.

For example, take the case of 23-year-old Erika, fresh out of nursing school, who's recently started her career as an Emergency Department (ED) nurse at a hospital in Florida. She quickly realizes the pace and acuity of the ED is too much for her. She's stressed out, anxious, and tired, and she's beginning to dread her shifts. She still loves nursing and wouldn't dream of leaving her career, but she sees the ED isn't a good fit. An older colleague suggests she speak with nurses from different specialties to see if another unit might be better aligned with her skills.

After looking into nursing duties across different departments, Erika decides to try the psychiatric unit. She finds the pace and demands are just right for her strengths and personality. She's able to transfer there, and she fits right in. Her stress levels dramatically reduce, and it's easy for her to recover from an intense shift or two over the weekend.

Fast-forward 15 years. If Erika finds she can't handle her job or her stress levels are higher than usual, that could be the beginning of burnout. When your beloved profession seems more like a burden than a calling, burnout might be to blame.

Here's some good news: Studies suggest that early career burnout doesn't seem to lead to any significant, negative, long-term consequences as long as it's handled. Burnout occurring later in a career might have more serious long-term effects—especially if it's left to linger without being addressed.

So, you might ask, *if medical providers are so burned out, why do we keep pushing?* Great question.

The truth is, there are plenty of reasons—many of which you can probably guess. For starters, we may be unable or unwilling to extricate ourselves from the comfort and security afforded by our professional track, such as tenure, pensions, benefits, or retirement perks. These dangling carrots can keep us hooked, making it hard to instigate changes despite clear signs of burnout. We might also feel pressure to remain committed to our profession, feel obligated to stay at a job where we help others, or find ourselves addicted to the success of our career path.

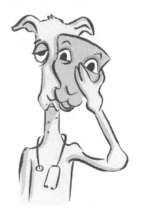

As a result, burned-out staff who are unable to create a physical boundary by changing jobs or taking time off from clinical practice often withdraw psychologically instead. This can lead to reduced empathy or an inability to express compassion, which in turn makes it more difficult to connect with patients or pick up on subtle symptoms or changes. It also depletes mental clarity, leaving medical practitioners more prone to error. In addition, burnout leads to higher levels of regret for having chosen medicine as a career. What a disastrous cycle to get caught up in!

—————

Burnout can masquerade as numerous other mental and physical conditions, but here are key symptoms to look for:

- **Depersonalization:** This symptom, in which a healthcare professional meets their patients with cynicism and callousness, should be a big red flag to physicians and caregivers who are drawn to their work precisely because of their desire to care for others.

- **Exhaustion:** There's the feeling of being tired at the end of a long workday, and then there's exhaustion—where sleep doesn't refresh you, your energy crashes sooner than expected, or you find yourself constantly tired no matter your sleep, eating, or exercise habits.

- **Apathy:** Feelings in burnout can range from recurring sadness to extreme irritability to a loss of interest in activities. It can show up as trouble concentrating, feelings of worthlessness, or at its most dangerous: thoughts of self-harm or suicide.

- **Anxiety:** It's normal to worry about things from time to time, but if worry persists or leads to panic attacks, it becomes an anxiety disorder. Anxiety can also manifest as intrusive thoughts; may incite an avoidance of situations and people; and can include physical symptoms like sweating, shortness of breath, rapid heartbeat, and other hyper-activation of the nervous system.

- **Dread:** You once looked forward to going to work or seeing patients, and now you feel reluctant, unwilling, or dread the work day.

- **Irritability:** An occasional lack of tolerance that manifests in a cranky mood is normal, but if you find that you're consistently irritable with patients or colleagues and/or at home with family and friends, there's a good chance burnout is the cause.

- **Impatience:** Impatience and irritability often go hand in hand when burnout sets in. Where once you had all the patience you needed for aspects of your work, as well as for your social life, now you find yourself snapping, easily frustrated, and annoyed by regular interactions.

- **Lack of will to work:** Often accompanying or prefacing depression, you may suddenly find that you don't have the will to get up and go to work each day. This feeling may not fully manifest as depression or dread, but you may find yourself dragging your proverbial feet, taking longer to get into work, even running late.

- **Sleep disturbances:** Trouble falling asleep, or waking up not feeling refreshed, is often an early sign.

- **Loss of appetite:** Lack of pleasure in eating is often one of the first signs that there's something going on psychologically. Since burnout is different for everyone, before you notice your feelings, you may notice a change in your eating habits.

- **Craving comfort food:** Likewise, if you find yourself eating even when you're not hungry or bingeing on sugary or salty foods, you may be trying to give your body a shortcut to the energy that's being drained.

- **Body aches and pains:** If you're experiencing an unusual amount of discomfort that seems unrelated to any health condition, pay attention. Often, people in a state of burnout stop exercising and don't engage in healthy self-care, which can worsen this symptom.

- **Using drugs, alcohol, and other substances as a replacement for energy and health:** When we have trouble managing the energy to work, many people turn to "easy" fixes: alcohol, sugar, caffeine, illicit substances, and junk food. If you notice you're drinking every night or picking up fast food on the way home because cooking feels like too much work, this can be a symptom of something bigger.

BURNOUT CAN MASQUERADE AS NUMEROUS OTHER MENTAL AND PHYSICAL CONDITIONS

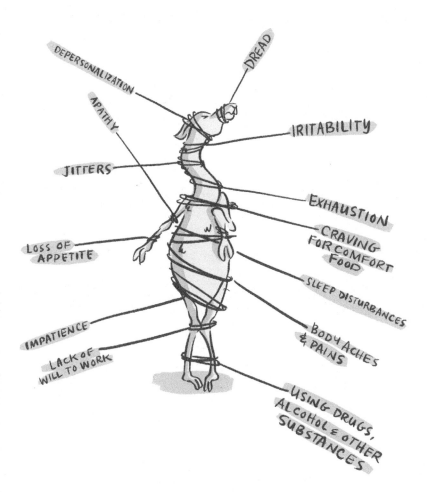

While this may look like a comprehensive list, burnout is personal and affects people in different ways. Regardless of how it manifests for you in particular, any of these symptoms (or others that suggest you're no longer thriving) should be considered potential warning signs that you're currently in or are headed toward burnout.

"Burnout occurs when your body and mind can no longer keep up with the tasks you demand of them."

— Del Suggs, Truly Leading

CHAPTER 3

A Ripple Effect: What Causes Burnout?

C ommon sense tells us that healthcare workers who are fulfilled at work and who experience a strong sense of purpose, satisfaction, and self-efficacy are in the best position to practice the art of medicine at its optimal level. Additionally, happy and healthy physicians and other caregivers are the ideal people to address the many problems within healthcare systems that lead to burnout.

What's tricky about this situation is that an abundance of fulfilled caregivers is not the current state of medicine—burnout is. Recent research shows that individuals are exiting their careers in medicine faster than they enter. Despite some organizational initiatives to reduce burnout, physician wellness expert Dr. Tait Shanafelt indicates that not only is the burnout epidemic getting worse, it's spilling out of healthcare institutions into the personal lives of physicians and caregivers, who are also reporting poor work-life balance.

While discussing job challenges with a pulmonologist friend of mine, Daniel, he confides that his wife has started to notice something alarming: "She told me I'm more burned out now than I was as a resident," he says.

He can't deny it—she's right.

"Truth be told, I was more satisfied with my work when I was a resident," he admits. Now he finds himself tired in a different way than the temporary fatigue that follows a long day at work in his Michigan clinic. "After thinking about it, I don't really like the person I've become in this role," he tells me. "Too much of my time is spent away from the part of this job I love most—direct patient care." He thinks he's become colder and more callus, and this is a painful discovery for him to reconcile.

Daniel's aloofness comes from feeling devalued. He no longer believes he's practicing cost-effective, patient-centered care. Instead, his work has become a series of hassles that includes relentless interference from insurance companies demanding complex prior authorizations and excessive documentation for billing purposes to avoid litigation threats. His on-call schedule, in conjunction with attempting to meet impossible panels of new patients, has become "ridiculous," and numerous other inefficiencies are slowly turning his beloved profession into a daily struggle.

Daniel's experience isn't unique. In fact, it's reflected across the entire healthcare industry—which is probably what led you to pick up this book.

Physicians enter clinical practice in good health, experiencing low rates of burnout and depression, and with fewer leading risks of death (such as cancer and cardiovascular disease). This doesn't last, though. Once they begin to practice, according to research from Mayo Clinic, long hours and chronic stress can cause physicians' work-life satisfaction to drop.

A report from Shanafelt et al examines 2014 survey data from nearly 7,000 U.S. physicians and compares it with the general population of working adults. The widening gap between the two groups is alarming—reporting doctors registered a work-life satisfaction of 40.9%, compared to 61.3% for those working outside of healthcare. One critical factor may be a high state of ongoing stress and the impact this has on an individual's emotional exhaustion. While 43% of practitioners reported meeting the criteria for emotional exhaustion, the same was true for only 24% of the general population. These effects compound, increasing the threat of workplace burnout. Only 28.4% of the general population believed they might have symptoms of burnout, whereas the same was true for 54.4% of physicians. In turn, this can elevate incidences of depression and even increase risk of suicide.

Daniel isn't alone in his struggle. Stricken by burnout, many doctors and nurses fake enthusiasm on the job while quietly praying they don't make a mistake that affects patient care or further burdens their colleagues.

An internist colleague of mine, Tamara, knows something is wrong one day when she finds herself talking with a patient who's struggling with a major illness. She later shares with me, "Here's this woman dealing with her mortality and in the moment, I didn't actually feel any empathy—I just forced a concerned expression onto my face and said the words I knew I was supposed to say."

She soon realizes this sense of depersonalization has been going on for some time. Burnout found her, and she knows she'll have to take some steps to alleviate it—it isn't going to get better on its own.

The problem of burnout is deeply entrenched in the culture of medicine itself. For one thing, physicians, nurses, and other clinicians are trained to put self-care as a priority of last resort. Medical school often teaches clinicians to be stoic and suck up their suffering.

However, the current epidemic isn't merely a product of care providers' personal tendency toward stoicism. These individuals have been heavily impacted by significant changes to the healthcare system overall. The addition of numerous burdens and hassles, increased administrative duties, and more time spent on computers dealing with quality measures and insurer requirements are all directly linked to a reduction in fulfillment and professional autonomy.

Healthcare Providers Are Like Camels

A good way to look at how this issue is affecting healthcare providers is through a familiar fable that illustrates burnout's cumulative impact. Using the concept of the straw that broke the camel's back, physician executive Dr. Paul DeChant writes:

Its owner, in an effort to transport as much straw as possible, keeps piling more and more on the camel's back. Camels are strong and can handle a lot. But at some point, even the strongest camel will buckle if enough weight is piled on.

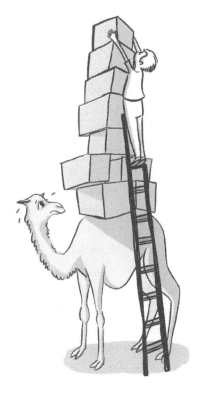

Just like the camel, as more and more responsibilities are piled on a physician or caregiver's plate, even the strongest and most passionate person will eventually begin to collapse beneath the weight.

Before you assume that the typical wear and tear of your job and its related stresses are burnout, let's take a look at the two main factors that stack up to create the problem of overloading: the job itself and the system or organization the job is part of.

The Job

The work environment (hospital or clinic) itself is a risk-factor for burnout. When you're in a service industry where you are constantly exposed to illness, trauma, and death, your own sensitive system eventually begins to wear down, even though it isn't happening directly to you. Even in a well-run organization, the nature of the work can be a source of fatigue. Over time, without intervention or self-care, burnout develops.

I know all too well how easily stress can negatively impact a physician or caregiver's health. When I'm in the midst of a critical-care situation, my heart rate rises, my breathing speeds up, my muscles tighten, and my palms glaze with sweat. These physiological responses only worsen the more critical the patient becomes. Repeat this reaction a few times a day for several days in a row, and the body takes a hit. Lack of concentration, restlessness, poor judgment, and insomnia become consistent. If this cycle continues, my health tanks.

Similarly, if your job involves prolonged hours tending to people who are grappling with intense conditions, such as drug addiction or domestic violence, it eventually takes a toll on your own mood and psyche. Anyone with an empathetic spirit will be affected by the pain of others over time.

The same is true if you're a caregiver to a parent who's been diagnosed with dementia, Parkinson's, or another degenerative disease that may require ongoing care or changes the person you knew. These forms of caregiving can sometimes feel thankless and exhausting.

First responders and people who work in caregiving fields, particularly palliative care and hospice work, are also especially prone to compassion fatigue and emotional strain. This is a response to working with individuals who are dealing with the consequences of traumatic events or incurable illnesses.

All of these roles are ones in which you're expected to be dynamic, productive, well prepared, and, most importantly, polite at all times—regardless of the situation. Compassion fatigue tends to have a rapid onset, whereas burnout is cumulative, but it can co-exist with burnout and even precipitate it.

The System

Healthcare organizations are also undergoing challenging times. The climate of healthcare includes steep price competition, narrower insurance networks, and a higher number of patients paying a larger amount of out-of-pocket expenses due to high deductible plans. All of these factors have added up to declining reimbursements. At the same time, administrative burdens on medical staff continue to increase. To solve these problems, hospitals and medical practices place greater pressure on physicians and nurses to do more with fewer resources. With national shortages in both physician and nurse populations, many hospitals are finding it difficult to stay adequately staffed.

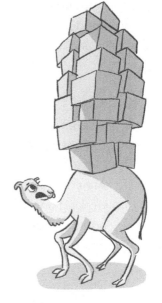

And that's not all. Additional threats to healthcare organizations include mergers and acquisitions, which may endanger existing fair contracts and the fate of these institutions in the long run. Newer quality metrics and requirements at the federal level also mandate already overburdened care providers with spending more time and energy on tracking and reporting issues of quality and safety.

In many ways, the system grinds down perfectly good practitioners. Hundreds of years ago medicine was a calling, not a "job." Given the dramatic ways the profession has changed over the years, from burdensome regulations to complicated payment structures to challenging workplace culture, it may not even be the same job you started out in decades ago.

While many of these changes are necessary for patient safety or for efficient reimbursement from insurance providers, overwhelmed staff experience burnout as they go to heroic lengths to survive a work environment that's brimming with barriers and frustrations. By often putting our own needs and self-care aside in the process, it's no wonder so many healthcare workers are breaking down physically and mentally.

∞

Here are seven questions to ask yourself to see if your job environment might be contributing to your burnout:

1. Are you pulling too many 10- to 12-hour days in a row or working on weekends? Do the demands of your extended hours or other job duties interfere with your relationships or leisure time?

2. Do you have vague or unclear directions about your role?

3. Are your decision-making abilities questioned or curbed, or do you lack a say in key job aspects, such as your schedule and vacation time?

4. Do you contend with poor communication, bullying behavior, or colleagues who compete with or undermine your work?

5. Do you work in a toxic environment where you experience isolation and lack of connection with colleagues?

6. Have you noticed a difference in values (purpose, ethics, and recognition) between you and leaders at your organization?

7. Has your work environment become more intense or acute than what you're accustomed to?

Digitization's Contribution to Burnout

Another major cause of burnout started with good intentions—technology, particularly Electronic Health Records (EHRs). In the past decade, for easier access to information and to centralize health data, physicians have been encouraged (and eventually required) to use EHRs.

There are clear benefits to EHRs for patients and medical professionals, but there are significant drawbacks, too. Technology was supposed to make the job easier, but research shows it's actually a huge source of physician and nurse frustration, as well as a leading factor in burnout.

A study published in *Health Affairs* reported that from 2011 to 2014, physicians began to spend increasing amounts of time engaged in "desktop medicine," which takes away time from face-to-face patient care. Another study found that the percentage of physicians reporting burnout increased over the same period; by 2014, more than half said they were affected.

While there's only a positive correlation between the data for now, there are other factors that may contribute to technology's negative impact. These include the learning curve providers experience as they contend with new systems and methods of charting patient information; how much extra time EHRs and other technology adds to an already packed workday; and the way "desktop work" pulls physicians away from patients. Whatever the reason, this is a topic that deserves continued attention.

We're still in the initial phases of the digitization of medical records, which means there are kinks to work out. We'll have to wait for the point in the future when functionality, accessibility, and transparency have improved to realize technology's true potential. Until we reach that stage, we have to endure, which means finding healthy ways to deal with the stress of these growing pains.

All these additional tasks beyond direct patient care may seem reasonable at the time they're introduced individually to a care provider's load. Cumulatively, however, they carry an enormously heavy weight that becomes too great a burden. Like our fabled camel, physicians begin to weaken under the increased load.

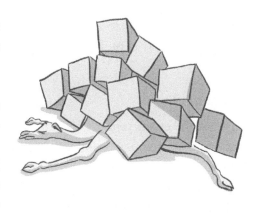

Physicians and nurses have breaking points—reaching the "last straw" when expectations and burdens become too high. In the same way we have to give the overwhelmed camel a rest, we've got to stop burdening physicians, caregivers, and other service workers.

Does Success Protect Against Burnout?

You might think: *I'm incredibly good at my job, and successful, too. Surely I can't be burned out?* Sadly, successful people can still burn out, and they may actually be more predisposed to burnout due to the likelihood they're going the extra mile in every area. In fact, recent psychological research suggests that even employees who are highly engaged in their work are at risk of burnout.

Everyone defines success differently. It's easy if you work in a high-pressured, competitive environment to believe that working 70 hours a week is a sign of success even when it leaves you fatigued and drained with little time for rejuvenation. Perhaps you feel pressure to take on multiple responsibilities to prove your worth. Laura Empson, author of *Leading Professionals: Power, Politics, and Prima Donnas*, observes that sometimes insecurity may be driving professionals to act in ways they think are successful, but which are actually contributing to eventual burnout.

—∞∞∞—

Burnout is characterized by emotional exhaustion, negative feelings about yourself and others, and a diminished sense of self-worth.

Ask yourself these three specific questions to assess your emotional health:

1. Do you feel burdened by the next task at work (despite support from staff)?

2. Do you feel your tasks lack purpose? For instance, do you feel like your patient is just another item on your checklist?

3. Is your inner voice consistently telling you, *I can't give anymore*, or, *I can't stand the people or circumstances at this job*?

If you answered YES to any of these three questions, you're most likely burned out. It's time to rehabilitate yourself, which we'll discuss in later chapters.

—∞∞∞—

"Hello? Do you see me? I'm working as creatively as possible and you want more and more and I'm out of juice and if you send me one more email I'm going to walk into the ocean and swallow water."

— COLE HARMONSON, PRE MIDDLE AGE

CHAPTER 4

Solutions: Organizational Resilience

B y this point, we've discussed how to recognize burnout and what causes it. In the next two chapters, we'll focus on actions that can help eliminate burnout and improve professional and personal fulfillment.

Burnout is widespread and systemic, making it an issue that needs to be addressed at two levels: the organizational and the individual. This chapter will focus on improving organizational resilience, while the next chapter is dedicated to fostering personal resilience.

A typical healthcare worker spends about 40-45 hours per week at the hospital or clinic, with some working as many as 60 or 70 hours. If we assume there are about 90 available hours in a week (after subtracting time for sleep, running errands, making food, caring for your house, etc.), around half or more of that available time is spent at work. Since such a significant commitment is

37

provided to an organization, management should ensure they're not only offering financial support and treating employees fairly, but also that workers are spending their time in a meaningful and purposeful way.

Some institutions might argue that by giving a salary and benefits, they're already making an exchange for someone's time or service. But burnout is so prevalent it's becoming a public health crisis. An organization's social responsibility extends beyond providing basic restitution. As the management guru Peter Drucker advised 60 years ago, "Our society has become… a society of institutions. And when our organizations fail to be effective and responsible, terrible things rush in to fill the void." He went on to say that organizations should "identify and address" problems—like widespread burnout—as they arise.

An Organization-Wide Problem

Staff Attrition

As burnout runs rampant, healthcare systems lose a high volume of physicians and other medical workers. Whether through early retirement, hours cutbacks, or outright quitting, burnout takes a heavy toll on the healthcare workforce. The costs of replacing a physician or a nurse (a process that includes recruitment, onboarding, training, and lost patient-care revenue during the hiring process) are estimated to be two to three times an individual's annual salary.

Mayo Clinic's 2014 survey of nearly 7,000 U.S. physicians found that one in 50 had made plans to leave the field in the next two years, while one in five planned to reduce their clinical hours within the same timeframe. The physicians who self-reported as burned out were more likely than others to carry out their intentions to quit.

This wasn't the first survey with these findings, either. In a 2013 Stanford University study, researchers learned that physicians who were experiencing burnout were more than twice as likely to leave their organization within two years. Researchers estimated that, without some kind of intervention, this meant nearly 60 Stanford physicians had a departure on the horizon. They calculated the cost of recruitment for each replacement would range from $250,000 to almost $1 million, and the economic loss over that time period would total between $15.5 and $55.5 million.

When care providers exit the profession early due to burnout, this profoundly worsens shortages of physicians and other healthcare roles. Not only does this create a period of crisis at the organizational level, it also has a direct impact on patients' access to care.

Reduction in Care, Safety, and Satisfaction

Burnout also impacts the quality of patient care. According to research published in JAMA, physicians experiencing burnout are twice as likely to be associated with a lower quality of care. Patients feel the impact, too. Due largely to the depersonalization that can accompany burnout, these physicians are three times as likely to be rated poorly by patients. It's easy to understand why— no patient wants to be seen by a checked-out, burned-out doctor or nurse. In turn, these subpar patient experiences can create a negative feedback loop, exacerbating burnout.

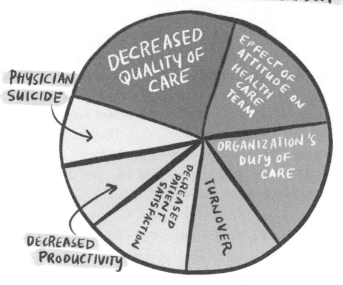

TOP REASONS TO ADDRESS PHYSICIAN BURNOUT

A burned-out workforce is likely to be less efficient and costlier when it comes to patient safety and satisfaction. In one study, researchers at the University of California, Davis reviewed literature to address how physician burnout affects quality and safety guidelines. They concluded that burnout of medical staff has a ripple effect throughout the entire healthcare system.

Looking to explore the effects of burnout on patient care, NIH researchers performed a meta-analysis investigating the quality and safety of patient care associated with physician burnout. Dr. Maria Panagioti and colleagues found that the best interventions came down to a dual approach, with a focus on changes at both the organizational and individual level.

Improving Organizational Resilience

Newer research indicates that 96% of executives, clinical leaders, and clinicians agree that burnout is a major problem among healthcare professionals.

Unfortunately, despite some organizational movement toward addressing burnout, most hospitals, medical centers, and practice groups are still approaching solutions as though they're purely the responsibility of the individual. While some organizations have already instituted or are encouraging wellness programs for physicians and other practitioners, certain stop-gap "solutions" such as stress-management workshops and seminars may simply add another task or role to a clinician's already overloaded plate—often barely making a dent in the reduction of burnout.

Many of these strategies bypass the root cause of the condition: organizational factors that are causing it in the first place. They're also often perceived skeptically by physicians as a band-aid solution to a larger problem. Additionally, by putting the onus exclusively on individuals, care providers may end up taking actions that provide personal benefit but are detrimental to the organization over time, such as reducing energy at work or cutting hours.

While it's great to see this long overdue attention to staff burnout and an increased focus on wellness, it's not going to solve the burnout crisis—at least not soon enough to help already distressed care providers. It's futile and even tragic to expect physicians, nurses, and other medical employees to heal themselves by marshaling "superhuman levels of resilience" when their work environments grow ever more burdensome.

Healthcare organizations have a responsibility to make changes from the top down that create a supportive practice environment and foster a culture of well-being. Beyond the organizational level, policy changes at the national level should be driving at least some of this change as well. At the same time, changes also need to be made from the bottom up, encouraging physicians and other clinicians to bolster their own resilience.

To do this, leaders should exhibit characteristics and skills that cultivate professional fulfillment and express a commitment to develop those skills in themselves and others when there are gaps. Based on Mayo Clinic research, I've outlined six organizational strategies that emphasize organizational resilience to address the problem of physician burnout.

1. **Recognize that burnout is a systemic issue**. Burnout is a combination of personal, organizational, and policy factors. While individuals absolutely can tackle burnout at a personal level, it doesn't stop the problem at its source. If an organization faced a different kind of large-scale threat to employee satisfaction, patient satisfaction, and quality of care, they'd scramble to develop a response, right? The same effort and resources should be put toward reducing burnout and promoting care provider engagement.

2. **Promote a culture of efficient leadership.** A supervisor's leadership skills carry a lot of weight. In fact, a 2013 study of more than 2,800 physicians at Mayo Clinic found that as the leadership skills of a physician's immediate supervisor increased, the likelihood of physician burnout decreased and physician satisfaction improved. When leaders are

effective, the benefits are far-reaching—impacting physicians and other staff, and extending all the way down to patients.

Effective leadership is a multi-step process. It starts with choosing leaders who have the ability to engage, listen to, develop, and lead physicians. Next, keep in mind that even natural leaders should be trained for their role. Finally, the individuals who are directly impacted by someone's leadership should be included in that person's performance assessment. Many healthcare organizations assess their leaders on overall performance targets, which can leave holes when it comes to determining efficacy.

Of course, leaders should also encourage staff to practice self-care and resilience. They should discourage the old model of thinking that physicians and other caregivers should be stoic, or that there isn't enough time to balance both patient care and physician/provider self-care. Leaders shouldn't be afraid to lean on external resources (like referrals to wellness programs or retreats) if they're unable to handle this element all on their own. Toward the end of this chapter, I've included examples of some healthcare organizations that are taking steps in the right direction when it comes to tackling burnout.

3. **Measure progress**. It's incredibly important to track and assess the performance of any initiative to improve burnout. Many organizations, such as the American Medical

Association, Mayo Clinic, and Stanford University, are developing new metrics to measure factors like resilience, joy in medicine, well-being, and more. If we don't keep track of our progress, how do we know if the changes we're making are having the right impact?

4. **Implement targeted solutions.** Organizations need to find specific ways to improve inefficiencies and create benchmarks to measure changes and improvements. Specificity is important when creating solutions to tackle burnout, especially because inefficiency is a primary cause of frustration in the practice environment. The reasoning is pretty obvious—when solutions aren't targeted, it wastes time and resources, which only adds to the frustration physicians and other care providers may be feeling.

If you're a healthcare change-maker or oversee decisions for a healthcare team, there are steps you can take to ensure your actions will really lessen burnout.

If you're in a healthcare leadership role, before you implement any changes, ask yourself these three questions:

1. Will this change ease the work burden for our overloaded healthcare providers?

2. Will this change lead to measurable improvement in quality or convenience for the people we serve?

3. Is there a revenue stream and additional staff to support the work involved in this change?

If you can't answer YES to these questions, you may need to pause and rethink what you're doing, or enlist a consultant who specializes in creating workplace efficiency or in meaningfully reducing employee burnout.

5. **Cultivate Community**. One of the most important elements in navigating the challenges of a healthcare provider role is peer support. Healthcare is a unique profession in which practitioners often work extended hours while dealing with extremely intense situations, as I discussed in Chapter Three. Care providers can't be expected to bear these burdens alone.

   A 2012 randomized trial from Mayo Clinic found that when physicians were given an hour of protected time every other week to meet with their colleagues *and* discuss the experiences of their job, it reduced burnout and improved meaning in their work. Can you guess which element of this experience was the most critical? It was the community. According to the study, "Participants in the facilitated small-group intervention experienced significant improvements in meaning, empowerment, and engagement in work beyond that seen in the physicians receiving only protected time."

6. **Provide flexibility and work-life integration**. If care providers are already burned out, they need to be able to seek changes that will allow schedule flexibility, whether that means working part-time or even starting shifts at a different time. Managers must be willing to work with staff one-on-one to make meaningful changes that facilitate work-life integration.

Physicians are hit especially hard by work-life integration challenges—reporting nearly twice the dissatisfaction around this issue as other U.S. workers. Physicians' long and grueling hours account for a significant part of this problem—approximately 45% of physicians work 60 or more hours per week. With such a high workload, it's challenging for physicians to integrate their personal and professional lives—a major factor in burnout.

For nurses—62% of whom work in the arduous environment of hospitals—issues of staffing, mandatory overtime, and workplace safety are the top three concerns related to work-life balance. Nurses are often required to work overtime and have little control over their schedules. High nurse-to-patient ratio is a major risk factor for burnout and on-the-job injuries as well.

Many other kinds of care providers or service professionals such as social workers and care coordinators also struggle with long hours and intense workloads. In many cases, either they don't have a direct superior or avoid appealing to their managers and leaders to intervene—most often due to concerns that to complain would jeopardize their jobs.

Part of the solution to burnout is to allow individuals to tailor their work hours so they can make time for other obligations. Reducing work hours is one evidence-based method for helping physicians recover from burnout (though it doesn't solve the organizational problems). While not every practice, hospital, or home can allow for care providers to reduce hours, organizations that are committed to reducing and preventing burnout will need to find creative workarounds to full-time (or overtime) schedules. With physician and nurse shortages predicted (and already in motion) for the next decade, creating more part-time positions within healthcare may become a necessary strategy.

What could be even more important than allowing physicians and other care providers to reduce their hours is to allow them flexibility in choosing when and how they work. Some may prefer to arrive at work later in the day or to work some longer days and some shorter ones throughout the week. This kind of flexibility acknowledges the preferences and limitations of individuals (especially working parents), and it's one way to circumvent a reduction in total hours while still offering employees a sense of control over their own schedules.

Additionally, organizations need to look closely at benefits such as vacation time and family leave. In lieu of work-hour reduction, other forms of compensation can be used, such as paid time off for professional development, service work, or the birth of a child. It's also important that physicians and other staff feel entitled to actually make use of their earned time off.

One area of need noted by many healthcare workers is the availability of a quality, affordable daycare located within or in the vicinity of their hospital or place of work. Accessible childcare enables practitioners to be more mentally present while providing patient care, and on-site childcare would also facilitate greater flexibility for coverage during delays or emergencies (such as when a surgery runs long). This is one work-life integration hospital administrations should seriously consider providing to their staff.

These organizational changes won't take place overnight, and some are easier to implement than others. But to meaningfully impact staff burnout, steps need to be taken at the organizational level to change the system in which care providers work.

Engagement and the Bottom Line

When physicians and other practitioners don't feel supported by their healthcare organization, everything suffers: professional

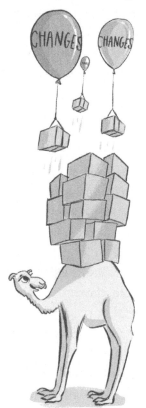

satisfaction, patient care, and the bottom line. As illustrated in this chapter already, there are multiple steps that hospitals, medical practices, and other healthcare environments can take to make positive change for providers, patients, and the organization's revenue—a win-win for all parties.

Employees' welfare is critical to a well-oiled healthcare machine. This is an area that organizations are going to have to take seriously if they hope to solve the burnout epidemic and leave patients feeling satisfied regarding their care.

Loneliness and isolation are key contributors to burnout, so one solution may be to increase physician engagement. (However, it's important to remember that even engaged physicians can experience burnout unless supported by other measures mentioned here.) Engagement has other benefits too: Gallup found that physicians who were fully engaged in their work had a 26% increase in productivity compared to physicians who were not engaged or who were actively disengaged while on the job. Engagement improves connection between care providers and patients, which in turn translates to better patient satisfaction and ultimately personal fulfillment.

As far as an organization's bottom line is concerned, simply by improving physician engagement health systems have been able to reap nearly half a million dollars in revenue per physician per year. And that's not all. Strategies that support and encourage physician engagement also increase revenue and corporate growth in other ways, too. Further study found that physicians who were fully engaged sent their hospital an average of 3% more outpatient referrals and 51% more inpatient referrals than disengaged physicians.

Gallup's analysis concludes that four key organizational approaches are responsible for successful physician engagement:

1. **Take a proactive and solution-oriented approach to physician problems,** especially those related to health reform changes.

2. **Focus on efficient communication** between physicians and system administrators.

3. **Support physician engagement** with hospital administration and ensure physicians' opinions are heard.

4. **Foster opportunities for professional growth**. For example, hospitals can promote physicians' expertise by publicizing them as speakers in their community or by providing new physicians with a mentor.

These measures can be applied to nurses, social workers, and other care providers as well. By adopting these four strategies (and others like them), healthcare organizations can go a long way toward building engagement, which pays dividends in all areas of growth.

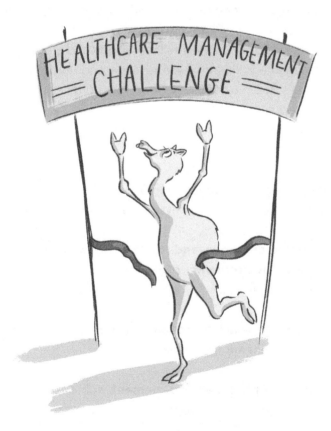

Resources for Implementing Meaningful Change

With a burnout epidemic on hand, how are leaders and managers responding in our organizations? The good news is, there's a small wave of change already taking place. According to Health Affairs, in 2016 the CEOs of 10 leading healthcare organizations met at the American Medical Association (AMA) headquarters in Chicago and made a commitment to prioritize the prevention of burnout by treating it as an urgent problem. They came up with an 11-pronged plan that includes adopting burnout measures, instituting team-based methods of care, encouraging government regulators to rethink the way they make rules, and spreading knowledge about the perils of provider burnout to other healthcare CEOs around the country.

Existing resources can help bring these changes to fruition. The AMA created the Steps Forward program, a series of online resources and tools dedicated to helping physicians tackle burnout, and individual solutions are popping up out of necessity in healthcare systems and practices around the country.

Academic institutions like Mayo Clinic and Stanford Health Care are paving the way for organizational intervention on burnout as well. Mayo Clinic has been at the forefront of research about the causes and severity of physician burnout and even created one of the first programs of its kind on physician well-being in 2007.

In 2017, the National Academy of Medicine (NAM), an independent organization comprising important leaders in health and medicine, convened an Action Collaborative on Clinician

Well-Being and Resilience to address burnout among physicians (and included nurses, mid-level providers, trainees, and other clinicians as well).

Other healthcare systems are following suit. North Carolina-based Novant Health spent more than $2 million getting a resiliency program off the ground to decrease burnout and increase well-being among its physicians, nurses, and administrative leaders. While over half of Novant's employed doctors have completed the voluntary wellness program since its launch in 2013, the organization is already seeing a benefit: "Those who participate in the program score higher—sometimes more than 50% higher—on key measures that include personal fulfillment, alignment with Novant's mission, and positive attitudes toward the organization," Fierce Healthcare reports. As a result, physician engagement for Novant Health's medical group is sitting in the 90th percentile nationwide.

Before healthcare reaches a point of no return, organizations and institutions across the country are going to need to pay close attention to these early adopters and begin implementing similar programs of their own.

Ultimately every manager has a choice to make. Do you want the people who work for your organization to feel overworked, mistreated, and undervalued, or do you want to foster an environment where your doctors, nurses, and other providers have an opportunity to work at their prime and serve proudly?

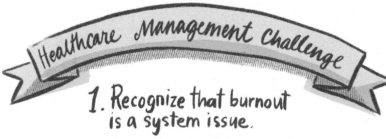

Healthcare Management Challenge

1. Recognize that burnout is a system issue.

2. Promote a culture of efficient leadership.

3. Measure it.

4. Implement targeted solutions.

5. Cultivate community.

6. Provide flexibility and work-life integration.

"Unwilling or unable to cut ourselves free of this modern machine we have built, we're dragged in its wake all too quickly toward our end. The virtue of a society's culture is reflected in the physical, mental, and emotional health of its people. The time has come to part ways with all that is toxic, and preserve our quality of life."

— L.M. BROWNING, SEASONS OF CONTEMPLATION

CHAPTER 5

Solutions: Individual Resilience

I n previous chapters we've looked at the organizational and social causes of burnout, as well as how to tackle them. We've discussed how to manage the outside element, including several ways to improve your professional environment and workflows at the institutional level. In this chapter, we'll focus on what changes we can make at the individual level to gain freedom from burnout.

Physicians and other healthcare providers are used to putting self-care on the back burner. Even after patient care is finished for the day, emails abound, voicemails stack up, and notes beckon. On top of this, like many areas of commerce, our entire healthcare industry is inundated by high-expectation performance measures and regulatory requirements.

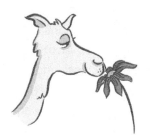

What this means is that most healthcare workers are simply trying to survive the day, rushing from patient to patient in an effort to stay accountable to the very institutions we've created. It feels like there isn't enough time or resources to facilitate the physical, emotional, and spiritual replenishing we need.

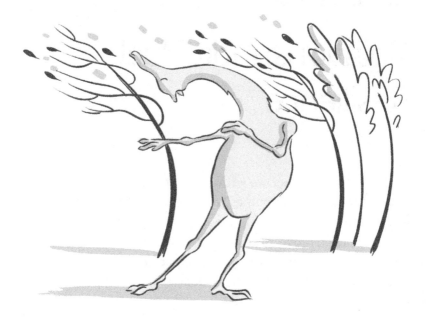

In this situation, freedom from stress and burnout can only be achieved through intentional, planned action and thought. By "freedom," I don't mean merely managing stress to a level that enables you to make it through the day. More significantly, freedom means cultivating joy in what you do. It means seeing happiness in those around you. It means looking out for one another and offering help when needed. It means being able to say no. It means having control over your schedule, living within a budget, and crafting a purposeful life. We'll see how to attain these goals in more detail in the following pages. The only prerequisite for this exercise is a commitment to engage in inner reflection.

Revisit the Nature of Your Job

Every field of human advancement requires innovation, which means we're faced with dynamic and changing work requirements. The moment we get comfortable in the present, we're thrown a new requirement to comply with or a new skill to master. In health-care, change stems not only from advances in medical knowledge, but also from outside forces such as digitalization, automation, and other technological progress and profit-driven motives.

Thriving in today's healthcare environment requires individuals to be flexible and adapt readily to the ever-changing workplace. To some, resilience comes naturally. It's an innate trait. For these people, it's easier to accept change and adapt quickly. But for many of us, resilience is an acquired skill.

Developing and fostering such resilience is the hallmark of some-one who maintains inner harmony. There's an abundance of research to support this. The American Medical Association has found that medical professionals who are resilient are both more prepared for the challenges of practicing healthcare and more likely to bounce back from burnout. Personal resilience also has a positive effect on the entire culture of your workplace.

Research shows that emotionally and physically healthy physicians, nurses, and other care providers tend to demonstrate and practice their values in a way that encourages similar positive behavior in their colleagues and patients. For this reason and others, healthcare institutions have an ethical responsibility to address burnout and make changes that will improve the health and career experience of practitioners. But even these changes may never achieve their desired potential—unless we're also making an earnest effort to find solutions that will allow us to be present and fulfilled rather than stressed, overburdened, and burned out. It's a huge responsibility, but with intention and care, you can achieve an inner transformation.

The path to recovering from burnout requires that you change the way you think about yourself and the world around you. The goal is to focus more on your experiences of enjoyment so that you gain a sense of gratifying participation in your job, home life, hobbies, and time spent with friends and family.

In the section that follows, I'll discuss three areas of your inner dimension that have the potential to make your life experiences not only optimal but, more importantly, enjoyable. They are:

1.   Finding meaning in your work.

2.   Managing leisure.

3.   Bringing order to the content of your mind.

Engage with Meaning in Your Occupation

For most of us, our occupation is the principal trade of our lives. To experience joy, it's important that you're able to engage with and derive meaning from your work. It's said that a smart person is one who gets paid for what she loves to do.

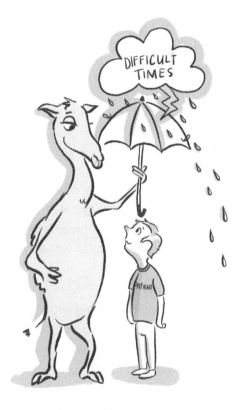

Observe these two scenarios to appreciate why *engagement with meaning* in your work is vital for a satisfying career.

Lacking Engagement in Work

Let's consider this first scenario, where your work has meaning, but you lack the engagement necessary to be satisfied.

We already know that a job as a healthcare provider has meaning in abundance—you alleviate the suffering of others with your skills and knowledge. But what if you're disengaged in the work you do or from the people who seek your care? Perhaps it seemed like the goal of meaningful work justified the effort it demanded at the outset, but as time has passed, you're finding that you don't (or can't) invest the same effort.

Lacking Meaning in Work

Now let's consider this second scenario, where you may be fully engaged in your work because it pays well, promises future savings, offers retirement benefits, provides material comforts, or affords a certain social status, all while lacking a higher meaning.

As a result, you may associate a price tag with every activity you do on the job. You may slip into thinking that being busy is more important and valuable than deriving joy from your occupation, and this can give you a sense of false worth. The busyness of work can even become addictive as you chase the next milestone. As busyness becomes your new identity, you may shame yourself for trying to make room for leisure. This can leave you feeling empty.

However, it's not as easy as it sounds to engage with meaning in your job, as there can be barriers to attaining this balance.

Let's examine three situations where optimizing engagement and meaning might be difficult.

1. You like what you do, but the "shadow work" is too much to handle. It's too stressful to continue, even though you love caring for your patients.

2. You like what you do, but you also have other interests outside of your profession, such as creating art, gardening, or riding horses. You're unable to balance your passion with your workload.

3. You used to like what you do, but not anymore. But you're far enough along in your career that you don't know what else you'd possibly do.

Now, let's explore these situations in little more detail.

Situation 1: Too Much "Shadow Work"

Shadow work is any added-on responsibility at your job that gets in the way of the heart of your work. While it may be necessary, it isn't pleasurable, even for someone who otherwise loves what they do. Former Harvard Magazine Editor Craig Lambert notes that, because of its repetitiveness and volume, shadow work is more than merely "a marginal nuisance snipping spare moments away from the edges of life." Shadow work occurs in plenty of professions (take teaching, for example), and medical practitioners aren't exempt.

Many healthcare workers grapple with decisions that are forced on them, that feel unfair, or that are institutionalized. Because so much of the job is dictated from above and is out of a provider's control, this can lead to considerable agitation.

Some of my colleagues (including Daniel, who you were introduced to in Chapter Three) wonder why they felt more fulfilled as residents or even in medical school than they do now, years away from those brutal training days. The reasons are twofold: If you follow a career path into medical or nursing school, the path is well lit. It's not easy, but the goals are clear and the boundaries are obvious. You receive frequent feedback and rewards. You also benefit from the closeness of your peers and the support of a tight-knit community during tough times. But real life is not always organized this way.

Instead, there are changing rules, hidden rules, and even rules that aren't fair. Our life experiences don't often reveal themselves to us all at once, the way the rules of standardized tests and board exams are clearly explained.

When you enter into the real job, the paradigm shifts. You have to learn to focus on experiences rather than accomplishments, such as passing an exam or graduating to the next level of a course. It's said that the end of all formal education is the beginning of a career that's motivated intrinsically. In this stage of your professional life, rewards are derived from seeing the person under your care receive quality treatment and (ideally) get better.

While the technical skills that *you*, as a physician, nurse, or other healthcare practitioner, have acquired are based on hundreds of years of research and experiments, patient care is not so technical. As care providers, we bring a great deal of ourselves to the work of medicine. The craft involves a significant amount of emotional labor, requiring empathy, presence, a clear head, and a compassionate heart. Anything—from a policy change to a new technical requirement—interrupts this flow, which can be a source of frustration and create resistance.

These are rarely the first things we think about when we consider the "job" of a physician, nurse, or healthcare worker. However, these ineffable parts of the role are what make us good at what we do, and it's also what makes us vulnerable to burnout.

The Solution for Too Much Shadow Work

If shadow work is burning you out, these three steps can help you optimize your work experience:

1. Acknowledge obstacles

2. List solutions

3. Pick the best option(s)

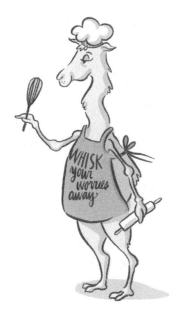

Acknowledge that your job has unwanted and unfavorable demands that are part of the organization or institution of healthcare as a whole. Start by admitting that you're unhappy or frustrated, that the outcome isn't what you wanted, and that you'd rather things were different. While you might have to come back to this step frequently for a while, don't let it interfere with the steps that follow.

For example, let's say a new requirement has been added to your already cumbersome charting for medical records. You feel burdened and angry that on top of your caregiving responsibilities, you now have to put in extra time to complete a task that shouldn't be yours in the first place.

Or, perhaps you're feeling resentful of a colleague who has a schedule that seems more optimal than yours. Your emotional state in this kind of situation contributes to burnout. Whether you use a journal to write down your feelings or talk through your emotions with a friend, family member, or therapist, take time to be honest with yourself.

Then, list all possible solutions. These solutions may be imperfect, but you still have to choose one. Using the examples above, you might begin to take note of the following: Is there an alternative to doing this task? Can you hand it off to someone else? Sometimes a scribe or medical assistant can take care of clerical tasks that distract from patient care, for example. Can you talk to your supervisor about streamlining this new requirement? Can you find a more efficient way to take care of it? Can you take the initiative to discuss a schedule change with your manager?

Finally, pick the best option. What should dictate your decision isn't the past, which is done and gone, but the future. Take a clear-eyed look at your available options. Which one will make you the happiest days or weeks or months in the future? Which one is the most effective? That's the one you should choose.

Once you select an approach to the problem or obstacle, commit to doing it to the best of your ability and to focusing on the positives.

While you work through these three steps, remember a few important things:

Continuous decision-making depletes will power. And when you lose will power, you lose self-control. Healthcare professionals make dozens of decisions throughout the day as they see their patients. If you've ever wondered why you binge eat junk foods or feel no interest in engaging in meaningful activities after going home from a long day at work, this is the reason—loss of will power and thus loss of self-control. It's helpful to take intermittent breaks during your work day. Whether you utilize a 10-minute guided meditation, a quick workout session, a brief walk outside of work, or even a short nap (if you're able to do so), re-invigorate by resting your mind and replenishing your will power.

Stop doing it all yourself. You've most likely heard the phrase, *You can't pour from an empty cup.* If you try to do everything yourself, you'll quickly find your internal resources drained, which makes you a much less effective care provider, as well as unhappy and burned out. It's common during medical or nursing training to try to become all things to all people in order to prove yourself. However, this attitude can carry over into your career, where it may be more difficult to delegate tasks or ask for help. Additionally, many individuals working in healthcare are overachievers who have a specific way of wanting things done. Be willing to let go of your vision of perfection in order to spread the work around appropriately.

Learning to delegate is a crucial step in strong leadership. If you're in a leadership role, know that good leaders learn to identify and communicate with the right staff or colleagues to share the weight of the workload. Sometimes, this also means you have to stand up to your own leadership and ask for better balance. Be sure you're not doing tasks that aren't within your work scope or compensation level.

Make sure major decisions about your job aren't made without you. You should be part of the important decisions that impact your job, regarding both your day-to-day workload and your long-term career trajectory. If decisions (especially ones that impose changes upon the way you do your job) are being made without you, speak up and say you want to be part of the decision-making process. And if you're the decision maker, make sure you involve the people who are directly affected by new changes.

Don't dwell on what you can't change. No matter how much you love your work, there are necessary duties that are simply cumbersome and unpleasant. Learn to identify what you can and can't change in your work environment. While you probably won't be able to choose your practice manager or avoid working with an EHR, there are always areas where you can offer your input and even drive positive change. Whether you join committees or express concerns to management, empower yourself to make change rather than dwell on what's out of your control. There's almost always something you can alter to improve your situation.

Support each other. Healthcare works best when we work together. Community is essential to a strong support network. The next time a colleague is feeling down about a patient outcome or a difficult situation, back them up, be a listening ear, or suggest resources that have helped you.

That being said, it's also important to identify the right people to talk to. Be sure your comments are being made to people who can take action, rather than venting about your frustrations or complaining without purpose. Be conscientious of your organization's hierarchy so you don't waste energy. Take the time to get to know leaders, managers, and administrators who are the most receptive, and make clear, solution-oriented suggestions for the best chance at a positive outcome.

Know when to move on. While most healthcare organizations look for ways to help their staff develop new skills to feel empowered, there are some environments that are truly unhealthy, emotionally toxic, or that don't support change. For instance, if you're giving input and it's ignored or not received well, if you feel sabotaged by colleagues or leadership, or if you've been disempowered, it may be a sign that your work environment is the cause of your burnout entirely, and you should look for a better place of employment. This is a heavy decision, so be sure you've really made every effort to ask for help or make changes.

Here's the bottom line: You have to use available resources to offload additional work, seek out ideas, simplify tasks, build a support network, and ask for help.

Situation 2: Balancing Work with Other Passions

One major cause of job dissatisfaction is that under the weight of mental and physical fatigue, people often put off doing the things they love. They bide their time, waiting for "someday" when they'll finally have time. This can be a problem. Let's use Anna's story as an example.

Anna is a 65-year-old Kentucky pediatrician closing in on retirement. For decades she's been looking forward to the point in her life when she can finally spend as much time as she wants riding her beloved horses—something she's barely been able to do with her demanding schedule.

Between patients, she occasionally finds herself daydreaming of being on horseback, the wind whipping her hair, breathing in the scent of fresh grass, the sun warming her shoulders instead of the fluorescent lights of the clinic and hospital.

Anna still loves her work, but she's put in more than three decades and is ready to indulge in her hobby.

Not long before retirement, Anna trips over the open dishwasher in her kitchen, falls backward, and injures her spine. She knows right away she's done something serious: the sudden weakness in her arms and the fierce pain in her neck and upper back are like nothing she's ever felt. She calls her husband to come home from work to take her to the hospital. It turns out she's sustained fractures in two of her cervical vertebrae.

A spinal surgeon overseeing her care recommends a rigid cast around her neck. It's going to take about three months for Anna's injury to heal, and surgery is possible. She's looking at a year or longer in physical therapy.

Once she's given her prognosis, Anna gets right to business: "How long until I'll be healed enough to ride my horses?" she asks.

The surgeon frowns. "I'm sorry, Anna, with an injury like this, horseback riding just won't be possible."

Anna is devastated. She spent her life putting off the one thing she wanted to do most, and now that she has the time, she no longer has the ability.

Anna recently relayed to me, "I learned the hardest lesson in the worst possible way: Don't put off what you love doing for later. If you don't make the time now, you may regret it."

The Solution for Balancing Personal Interests

It's easy to lose sight of our own needs and identity when we're deep in our work. *Make note of a few practical steps to take to keep this from happening.*

Schedule time for yourself. No matter how pressing your job needs are, create a personal schedule that includes things that are crucial to your mental and physical health, from sleep to exercise to leisure activities. Then stick to your schedule with as much commitment as you do your work obligations.

Prioritize activities. A healthcare professional might be "caring" for an ailing individual but is distracted by other personal

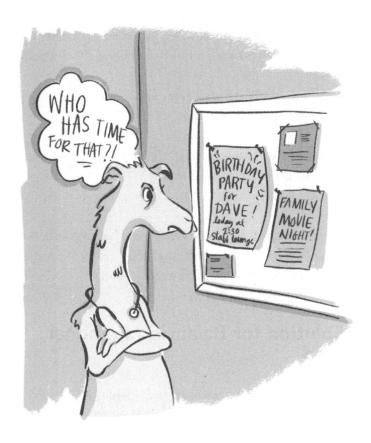

commitments. He might be worried about running late for the next patient or overwhelmed by patient notes. Or she may be spending her session concerned about not making it to her daughter's recital as planned. She may feel that she's always playing catch up, never present in the moment. By making time for what's important to you, you'll get more enjoyment not only out of your family activities or other passions, but you'll also perform better at work.

Manage leisure. When you're at work, you most likely look forward to getting home and taking advantage of your leisure time. Yet in many ways, jobs are easier to enjoy than free time because they have built-in rules and challenges, which encourage concentration and a more immersive experience.

Leisure time, in contrast, is unstructured and may even require effort in order to be enjoyed. Passive activities, such as watching TV or listening to music, might temporarily fill the time, but it's not the same as a hobby, which engages the spirit and heart.

Most jobs and many leisure activities—especially those involving the passive consumption of mass media—are not designed to make us happy and strong. Unless we take charge of leisure time, it's likely to be disappointing. Passive entertainment (especially habitual use) leaves us more drained and exhausted than before. We usually just pick up another form of entertainment until this runs its course. Then the cycle continues.

Without structure our minds wander, and it's extremely difficult to focus. We rely upon external stimulation and feedback to focus our attention instead. When that's lacking, our thoughts can become chaotic—resulting in a state of apathy. This apathy is a roadblock to productively balancing our professional lives with our personal ones.

Apathy should be an opportunity for re-creation. In his book *Flow*, psychologist Mihaly Csikszentmihalyi lists the essential steps to manage unstructured time:

1. Pick a hobby that gently challenges you. Set an overall goal, and as many sub-goals as are realistically feasible.

2. Find ways of measuring progress through feedback (your own and also others).

3. Concentrate on what you're doing, and make finer and finer distinctions in the challenges involved in the activity.

4. Develop the skills necessary to interact with the available opportunities.

5. Keep raising the stakes if the activity becomes boring.

People who learn to creatively manage their free time end up feeling that their lives have become more worthwhile.

Your hobbies don't have to be lofty, either. You might choose to spend your time running, learning a new language, pursuing an art form or a musical instrument, or figuring out how to bake a perfect pie (your neighbors may be especially grateful for this one).

Situation 3: You Feel Stuck in Your Career

It's easy to get comfortable with the status quo, even when that state of being is unfulfilling, unhappy, or stressful. If you've given change a few tries and it hasn't paid off, you might be tempted to stop trying. Instead, these situations call for courage to find new and innovative solutions to old problems.

Sometimes this means changing yourself in ways that may be new or challenging. Rather than being broken by what's difficult, look for ways to consciously step outside your comfort zone and seek change that will make things better for you and others. Don't listen to the voice inside that says an adjustment is too hard—sometimes the answer is to make your change even bigger and bolder.

The Solution for a Career Flatline

Most healthcare professionals come to their work as a calling. If you're feeling the symptoms of burnout begin to take hold, take some time to connect with what brought you to your field in the first place. This might be as simple as volunteering with an organization in your community that gets to the heart of what you love (or once loved) about your career.

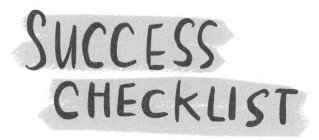

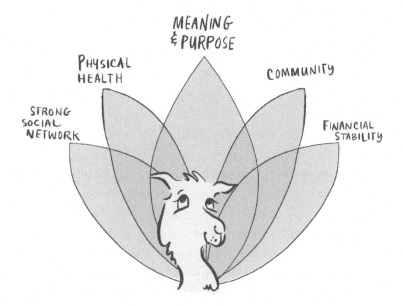

MEANING & PURPOSE

PHYSICAL HEALTH

COMMUNITY

STRONG SOCIAL NETWORK

FINANCIAL STABILITY

Don't let yourself become stagnant in your workplace. If you feel called to do more than see patients, find out if there are other growth opportunities or roles you can take on that accord with your sense of purpose. Stay mindful of how this impacts other areas of your schedule, though, including your time for resting and recharging. Don't exacerbate your burnout by adding one more thing to an already too-full plate.

You can deepen your connection to your daily habits and actions by checking in with yourself in a few key ways.

Identify your values. In your reflection time, think about and even write down your values and priorities at this particular point in your life. Is there a match between your values and your lifestyle? How about your values and your work? Look for places of misalignment and be courageous—take steps to make changes where necessary.

Learn to say no. One of the many contributing factors to burnout is being spread too thin. You may have too much going on in your life, which can take a mental and even physical toll. When you step back and set boundaries, you may also help others prioritize their own needs.

Make incremental lifestyle changes. Big changes may be out of your control or beyond your reach, but small changes are absolutely possible. For instance, if you wanted to lose weight, you'd focus on healthy eating and regular exercise and, if you're consistent, the process alone would enable you to reach you goals. Along the way, you'd also improve your health and feel better. This same idea can be applied to other goals as well. Remember, if you don't enjoy the journey, what's the point?

You have the power to change some of the unhappiness that gathers alongside burnout. You may have to leave the comfort zone of familiar practices that are no longer working for you—including habits, patterns, and relationships that seem comfortable by virtue of being what you've always known.

Your goal is to feel more alive and less attached to your worries—to break free from the patterns of your mind. To be able to do this is the hallmark of resilience.

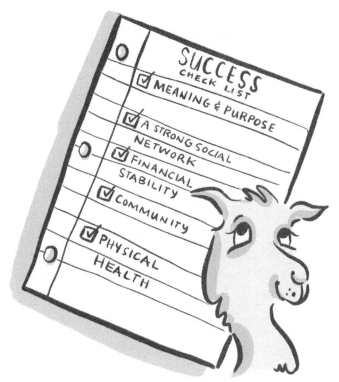

Are These Strategies Working?

Here's the litmus test: *Watch for FIR—frequency, intensity, and recovery time from emotional disturbances—such as dealing with stressors at work (or even at home).*

- Frequency: How frequently are you getting emotionally disturbed by something that takes place in your life (how often in a week or a day are you losing your cool)?

- Intensity: How strongly are you reacting to these situations?

- Recovery: How quickly are you able to bounce back to a state of calmness?

When looking for an end to burnout, remember that this is not a single-solution problem. You'll need to practice self-care, create new habits that shore up resilience, *and* seek support for positive changes from within your healthcare organization. While there are some challenges that can't be solved at the organizational level and will require legislative and institutional shifts over time, there's still plenty of action you can take on your own.

Taking steps at the personal level—both at work and at home—can make a significant difference in your burnout. These changes can go a long way in empowering you on your journey and helping you feel better.

NOTES ON SOURCES

CHAPTER ONE
BURNOUT: A KNOTTY PROCESS

1. "healthcare workplace is in a burnout epidemic": Shanafelt, T. D., Dyrbye, L. N., & West, C. P. (2017). Addressing Physician Burnout. *JAMA,317*(9), 901. doi:10.1001/jama.2017.0076

2. "In the United states": Lacy, B. E., & Chan, J. L. (2018). Physician Burnout: The Hidden Health Care Crisis. *Clinical Gastroenterology and Hepatology,16*(3), 311-317. doi:10.1016/j.cgh.2017.06.043

3. "more than 42% of physicians report": (n.d.). Retrieved from https://www.medscape.com/slideshow/2018-lifestyle-burnout-depression-6009235

4. "Germany, Hungary, the United Kingdom, Portugal": Sablik, Z., Samborska-Sablik, A., & Drożdż, J. (2012). Universality of physicians' burnout syndrome as a result of experiencing difficulty in relationship with patients. Archives of medical science: AMS, 9(3), 398-403.

5. "drive physicians to suicide": Physician Suicide. (2018, August 01). Retrieved from https://emedicine.medscape.com/article/806779-overview

6. "Nurse burnout is on the rise": Zimmerman, B. (n.d.). Survey: 70% of nurses report burnout in current position. Retrieved from https://www.beckershospitalreview.com/

human-capital-and-risk/survey-70-of-nurses-report-burnout-in-current-position.html

7. "one study found": Mudallal, R. H., Othman, W. M., & Al Hassan, N. F. (2017). Nurses' Burnout: The Influence of Leader Empowering Behaviors, Work Conditions, and Demographic Traits. Inquiry: a journal of medical care organization, provision and financing, 54, 46958017724944.

8. "as 43% of nurses and other caregivers": Dyrbye, L. N., Shanafelt, T. D., Sinsky, C. A., Cipriano, P. F., Bhatt, J., Ommaya, A., . . . Meyers, D. (2017). Burnout Among Health Care Professionals: A Call to Explore and Address This Underrecognized Threat to Safe, High-Quality Care. NAM Perspectives, 7(7). doi:10.31478/201707b

9. "A 2017 Stanford report": Retrieved from http://wellmd.stanford.edu/content/dam/sm/wellmd/documents/2017-ACPH-Goh.pdf

CHAPTER TWO
RECOGNIZING BURNOUT

1. "only about 9% of the physicians": Medscape National Physician Burnout & Depression Report 2018. (n.d.). Retrieved from https://www.medscape.com/slideshow/2018-lifestyle-burnout-depression-6009235?faf=1#17

2. "Studies suggest that early career burnout": Cherniss, C. (1992). Long-term consequences of burnout: An exploratory study.

Journal of Organizational Behavior, 13(1), 1-11. doi:10.1002/job.4030130102

3. "key symptoms to look for": Know the signs of job burnout. (2018, November 21). Retrieved from https://www.mayo-clinic.org/healthy-lifestyle/adult-health/in-depth/burnout/art-20046642

CHAPTER THREE
A RIPPLE EFFECT: WHAT CAUSES BURNOUT?

1. "Recent research shows" and "according to research from Mayo Clinic": Olson, K. D. (2017). Physician Burnout—A Leading Indicator of Health System Performance? Mayo Clinic Proceedings, 92(11), 1608-1611. doi:10.1016/j.mayocp.2017.09.008

2. "prone to compassion fatigue": Compassion Fatigue. (2017, January 04). Retrieved from https://www.stress.org/military/for-practitionersleaders/compassion-fatigue/

3. "A study published in *Health Affairs*": Penson, D. F. (2018). Re: Electronic Health Record Logs Indicate that Physicians Split Time Evenly between Seeing Patients and Desktop Medicine. Journal of Urology, 199(1), 20-20. doi:10.1016/j.juro.2017.09.105

4. "Another study found that": Penson, D. F. (2016). Re: Changes in Burnout and Satisfaction with Work-Life Balance in Physicians and the General US Working Population between 2011 and

2014. Journal of Urology, 195(5), 1568-1568. doi:10.1016/j. juro.2016.02.051

5. "working 70 hours a week": Kaufman, S. B. (2014, July 23). Why Your Passion for Work Could Ruin Your Career. Retrieved from https://hbr.org/2011/08/why-your-passion-for-work-coul

CHAPTER FOUR
SOLUTIONS: ORGANIZATIONAL RESILIENCE

1. "physicians may be exiting their careers in medicine": Sinsky, C. A., Dyrbye, L. N., West, C. P., Satele, D., Tutty, M., & Shanafelt, T. D. (2017). Professional Satisfaction and the Career Plans of US Physicians. Mayo Clinic Proceedings, 92(11), 1625-1635. doi:10.1016/j.mayocp.2017.08.017

2. "becoming a public health crisis": Stressed in America. (n.d.). Retrieved from https://www.apa.org/monitor/2011/01/ stressed-america.aspx

3. "Mayo Clinic's 2014 survey": Sinsky, C. A., Dyrbye, L. N., West, C. P., Satele, D., Tutty, M., & Shanafelt, T. D. (2017). Professional Satisfaction and the Career Plans of US Physicians. Mayo Clinic Proceedings, 92(11), 1625-1635. doi:10.1016/j. mayocp.2017.08.017

4. "the cost of recruitment for each replacement": Paid Program: High Cost of Physician Burnout. (2018, February 02). Retrieved from https://partners.wsj.com/ama/charting-change/ stanford-physician-burnout-costs-least-7-75-million-year

5. "leadership skills carry a lot": Shanafelt, T. D., Gorringe, G., Menaker, R., Storz, K. A., Reeves, D., Buskirk, S. J., . . . Swensen, S. J. (2015). Impact of Organizational Leadership on Physician Burnout and Satisfaction. Mayo Clinic Proceedings, 90(4), 432-440. doi:10.1016/j.mayocp.2015.01.012

6. "2013 Stanford University study": Hamidi, M. S., Bohman, B., Sandborg, C., Smith-Coggins, R., Vries, P. D., Albert, M. S., . . . Trockel, M. T. (2018). Estimating institutional physician turnover attributable to self-reported burnout and associated financial burden: A case study. BMC Health Services Research, 18(1). doi:10.1186/s12913-018-3663-z

7. "According to research published in JAMA": Panagioti, M., Geraghty, K., Johnson, J., Zhou, A., Panagopoulou, E., Chew-Graham, C., . . . Esmail, A. (2018). Association Between Physician Burnout and Patient Safety, Professionalism, and Patient Satisfaction. JAMA Internal Medicine, 178(10), 1317. doi:10.1001/jamainternmed.2018.3713

8. "physician burnout affects quality and safety guidelines": Dewa, C. S., Loong, D., Bonato, S., & Trojanowski, L. (2017). The relationship between physician burnout and quality of healthcare in terms of safety and acceptability: A systematic review. BMJ Open, 7(6). doi:10.1136/bmjopen-2016-015141

9. "NIH researchers performed a meta-analysis": Wise, J. (2018). Burnout linked to suboptimal patient care, study finds. Bmj. doi:10.1136/bmj.k3771

10. "clinicians agree that burnout is a major problem": Why Physician Burnout Is Endemic & How Health Care Must Respond. (2017, December 01). Retrieved from https://catalyst.nejm.org/physician-burnout-endemic-healthcare-respond/

11. "make changes from the top down": Physician Well-Being: Efficiency, Resilience, Wellness. (2018, November 26). Retrieved from https://catalyst.nejm.org/physician-well-being-efficiency-wellness-resilience/

12. "six organizational strategies": Shanafelt, T. D., Gorringe, G., Menaker, R., Storz, K. A., Reeves, D., Buskirk, S. J., . . . Swensen, S. J. (2015). Impact of Organizational Leadership on Physician Burnout and Satisfaction. Mayo Clinic Proceedings, 90(4), 432-440. doi:10.1016/j.mayocp.2015.01.012

13. "a 2013 study of more than 2,800 physicians at Mayo Clinic": Shanafelt, T. D., & Noseworthy, J. H. (2017). Executive Leadership and Physician Well-being. Mayo Clinic Proceedings, 92(1), 129-146. doi:10.1016/j.mayocp.2016.10.004

14. "2012 randomized trial from Mayo": West, C. P., Dyrbye, L. N., Rabatin, J. T., Call, T. G., Davidson, J. H., Multari, A., . . . Shanafelt, T. D. (2014). Intervention to Promote Physician Well-being, Job Satisfaction, and Professionalism. JAMA Internal Medicine, 174(4), 527. doi:10.1001/jamainternmed.2013.14387

15. "reporting nearly twice the dissatisfaction": Dyrbye, L. N., Shanafelt, T. D., Sinsky, C. A., Cipriano, P. F., Bhatt, J., Ommaya, A., . . . Meyers, D. (2017). Burnout Among Health

Care Professionals: A Call to Explore and Address This Underrecognized Threat to Safe, High-Quality Care. NAM Perspectives, 7(7). doi:10.31478/201707b

16. "62% of whom work in the arduous environment": Mullen, K. (2015). Barriers to Work–Life Balance for Hospital Nurses. Workplace Health & Safety, 63(3), 96–99. https://doi.org/10.1177/2165079914565355

17. "one evidence-based method for helping": Mullen, K. (2015). Barriers to Work–Life Balance for Hospital Nurses. Workplace Health & Safety, 63(3), 96–99. https://doi.org/10.1177/2165079914565355

18. "Gallup found that physicians who were fully engaged": Gallup, Inc. (2014, June 05). Want to Increase Hospital Revenues? Engage Your Physicians. Retrieved from https://news.gallup.com/businessjournal/170786/increase-hospital-revenues-engage-physicians.aspx

19. "and 51% more inpatient referrals" and "in 2016 the CEOs of 10 leading healthcare organizations": https://news.gallup.com/businessjournal/170786/increase-hospital-revenues-engage-physicians.aspx

20. "the Steps Forward program": Preventing Physician Burnout. (n.d.). Retrieved from https://edhub.ama-assn.org/steps-forward/module/2702509

21. "Fierce Healthcare reports": How Novant Health tackled physician burnout. (2018, May 08). Retrieved from

https://www.fiercehealthcare.com/practices/how-novant-health-tackled-physician-burnout-carl-amato

CHAPTER FIVE
SOLUTIONS: INDIVIDUAL RESILIENCE

1. "The American Medical Association has found that": Improving Physician Resiliency. (n.d.). Retrieved from https://edhub.ama-assn.org/steps-forward/module/2702556

2. "Research shows that emotionally and physically healthy physicians": Physician Well-Being: Efficiency, Resilience, Wellness. (2018, November 26). Retrieved from https://catalyst.nejm.org/physician-well-being-efficiency-wellness-resilience/

ACKNOWLEDGEMENTS

Heartfelt thanks to Jordan Rosenfeld for her help in developing the early manuscript and supplying valuable feedback. I'd also like to acknowledge creative illustrator Klay Arsenault for providing images that brought life to the subject of this book. Special thanks as well to Kirsten Clodfelter who was instrumental in shaping this book with a sharp eye and astute intellect. Without her masterful guidance and editing, this book wouldn't have been possible.

ABOUT THE AUTHOR

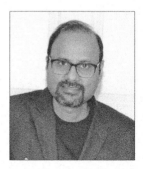 Rajeev Kurapati, MD is American Board Certified in Family Medicine and holds an MBA from the University of Missouri. He currently works as a full-time, hospital-based physician at a large healthcare system in Northern Kentucky. His writings pertaining to medicine, culture, and lifestyle have been widely published. He is the author of two award-winning books, *Unbound Intelligence* and *Physician: How Science Transformed the Art of Medicine*. Learn more at www.RajeevKurapati.com.